THE HEALING GARDEN

Also available from Grey House in the Woods

the Voice within the Wind
of Becoming and the Druid Way
Greywind

the Path through the Forest
a Druid Guidebook
Julie White & Graeme K Talboys

Arianrhod's Dance
a Druid Ritual Handbook
Julie White & Graeme K Talboys

Wealden Hill
a novel
Graeme K Talboys

Singing with Blackbirds
Stuart A. Harris-Logan

Inventing Reality
Tom Graves

Needles of Stone
Tom Graves

THE HEALING GARDEN

An Introduction To Herbs

Second Edition

NANCY BENCH

GREY HOUSE IN THE WOODS

Cover by Greywind
Photographs copyright Peter Bench

Cover pictures (from top to bottom): Squinancy, Borage, Evening Primrose, Nasturtium, Coltsfoot, Horehound.

Acknowledgements

I should like especially to thank Christine who has done the illustrations and deciphered my scribbles, and Peter who has been both helpful and patient. My thanks also to Barbara and Graeme for their faith in me, particularly to Graeme, a brilliant and helpful editor; without him nothing would have come to fruition.

The cover photographs were kindly supplied by Peter Bench.

CONTENTS

INTRODUCTION

I have been involved with plants for most of my life. The last thirty years have been spent at The Herb Nursery in Thistleton, Rutland – now run by my son and his wife.

My parents taught me the value of herbal remedies, dosing me with chamomile and other such things. My husband taught me to value the earth and all her goodness.

As a registered healer I am very aware of how people will differ in their reaction to any kind of therapy. A remedy that works well for one person may have either no effect at all or an unpleasant one on another, therefore caution and small doses at first are essential.

The plants in this book are not described in any detail, for with both common and Latin names given, they are easy to research to make sure that you have the correct one. As a lot of wild flowers have names that vary from region to region and country to country, knowledge of the Latin name is essential.

There is a mystique about herbs which can make people wary. At the nursery we grow decorative as well as useful plants; a comment which has been much enjoyed by us all was: 'I didn't know you grew plants as well!'

The most important factor in choosing is to use personal taste rather than book say-so; that is, after you are certain you know your plant. However, a good book such as those in the Bibliography at the end along with careful study of the plant should be enough.

A consideration of the plant's habits is needed. An annual plant has one season in which to produce flowers and seed to perpetuate itself, as with dill and coriander. A biennial will not flower until its second year after which it will set seed and probably die, as with parsley and evening primrose, although sometimes they live on for a further year. A perennial will send up shoots from its roots in spring, flower, and seed according to variety and then rest until the next year, as in sweet cicely and bistort.

Most of the plants mentioned are not particularly fussy about position, although generally they are happier if the soil is not too rich. If you keep them in pots go for a medium base; you can always use a foliar feed if needed. Do not use manure on herbs as it is too strong.

When considering shrubby plants, most of which are Mediterranean in origin (such as sage, thyme, rosemary, and lavender), well drained and sunny is the secret. These plants will succumb to wet feet rather than the cold.

If you have some leaves or flowers surplus to requirements, they can be dried. Most can be satisfactorily dealt with in an airing cupboard or similar warm place. Make sure the plant material is dry and free from pests. The best time to pick is on a sunny morning when the plant is rested after the night, but not touched by the hot sun later in the day.

Store dried material in a dark, dry place and use to make an infusion (also known as a tea or tisane). The standard measurement is 1oz dried herb to 1 pint of boiling water. Allow to stand and then strain, adding honey to taste. This will give 3 small cups which can be drunk as required.

A tincture is a preparation where the plant material has been preserved in alcohol. These are more usually prescribed by a herbalist. It is potent stuff and 5 to 10 drops in water is the usual dose.

Essential oils, used in aromatherapy, are not for internal use. Nor should they be used directly on the skin. They should be diluted in a carrier oil if used for massage. When added to a bath full of water, five drops is sufficient. The one exception is lavender, small quantities of which can be used without dilution.

If you are ever in doubt about any of these things, consult a qualified herbalist or aromatherapist. Better still; see if there are any reputable courses being held in your area.

THE
HERBS

Abscess Root
Polemonium reptans

With blue flowers and green leaves shading to bronze, this perennial makes an attractive garden plant. It is related to Jacob's Ladder *Polemonium caeruleum* – so called because its leaves are ladder-like in formation.

The ancient Greeks prescribed the *caeruleum* in wine for dysentery and poisonous bites and it passed into the European pharmacopoeias for use against rabies and syphilis. Both plants are sometimes called Greek Valerian although they are not related to the *Valeriana officinalis*.

Abscess Root, according to Mrs Grieve, is North American in origin, growing in damp woodlands and by riverbanks. Both species have similar properties and would have been of use both externally and internally for inflammatory and feverish conditions. They are seldom used today.

Aconite, Monkshood
Aconitum napellus

A tall, attractive, herbaceous plant which looks rather like a delphinium with deep blue, hooded flowers. It is one of the most toxic of plants and subject to legal restriction in some countries. It is as well to be aware of this. Although it can be of value to qualified practitioners and is beautiful to look at, there can be problems if it is handled frequently.

An indication of its toxicity can be seen from the frequency with which it appears as a poison in murder mystery novels. Agatha Christie used it several times and it is also featured as the title of one of Ellis Peters' Cadfael stories.

Agrimony
Agrimonia eupatoria

A perennial wild flower of medium height also known as Church Steeples because of its spikes of yellow flowers. The seed capsules are grooved and covered with small hooked spines.

A plant of hedgerows and railway lines, it used to be a common sight. From the time of the Saxons, or even before, it has been valued in producing a health giving tea in its own right as well as later being added to very expensive imported tea. The leaves have a faintly spicy odour of apricots, but to our modern taste are slightly bitter.

It contains a high proportion of tannins and so is useful for stomach upsets or as a soothing wash for skin eruptions. Its other main ingredient, silica, is a factor in its healing power and in the 15th century it was an ingredient in Arquebusade Water, a wash for gunshot wounds.

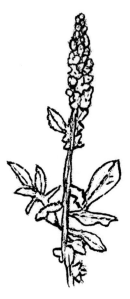

Alecost, Costmary
Tanacetum balsamita

A hardy, perennial herb growing 2 or 3ft high. A native of Asia, it found its way to England by the 16th century or possibly even earlier. It will grow anywhere, but prefers a dry position. The small flowers are yellow and daisy-like.

The spicy, rather sharp flavour was used as an addition when brewing, hence the name Alecost ('cost' being derived from the Latin *costum*, meaning 'aromatic plant'). The plant was also widely connected with the Virgin Mary during the Middle Ages, leading to the name Costmary.

It seems possible that another alternative name, Bible Plant, dates from the Puritan era and early American colonists who used the smooth, scented leaves as book-marks and reminders of home.

The leaves dried with rosemary and lavender will intensify the aroma of pot-pourri or will freshen a linen cupboard and help to deter moths. They were also used as a strewing herb, scattered on floors to help cleanse and sweeten the room, especially great halls where many people gathered to eat and sleep.

Culpeper used it as a tonic herb although it is not much used today. A bruised leaf rubbed on a bee sting is reputed to relieve the pain and a salve can be made with a suitable base to soothe burns and bruises. It has a strong flavour, but small amounts can be added to salads or cooked with chicken.

Camphor Plant
Tanacetum balsamita var. tomentosum

A herbaceous perennial which is happy in partial shade. A good addition to any large border. It is similar to Alecost, but used for its scent. It has smooth, grey leaves which smell strongly of camphor and pleasant, white daisy-like flowers. The leaves can be dried to go in a pot-pourri or tied in bunches with tansy and lavender or rosemary to hang in wardrobes to discourage moths.

Alexanders
Smyrnium olusatrum

A native plant of Macedonia, the country of Alexander the Great, this tall biennial was introduced into Britain by the Romans. It is also known as Black lovage as it is somewhat similar in flavour and habit to lovage, but the seeds are black.

One of many undemanding plants, it is both good looking and useful. The leaves are a deep green, tend to be shiny, and when still young can be added to salad or as flavouring to a white sauce. The stems can be cut and peeled like rhubarb and cooked as a vegetable. The young buds can be washed (if necessary) and cooked for a minute or two in boiling water with a pinch of salt. When cool, they can be added to an oil and vinegar dressing.

Lenten pottage contained a mixture of alexanders and nettle with, perhaps, watercress or chickweed. A pottage was originally porridge so the herb pottage would have a basis of oatmeal and water with the addition of whatever herbs were available, preferably finely chopped and added to the cooked mixture. During Lent, when diet was restricted, the Lenten pottage would have been welcome. A knob of butter and a pinch of salt, and maybe a thick slice of bread, would make a nourishing and filling meal.

Alkanet
Pentaglottis sempervirens

Also known as Anchusa or Bugloss, although the Viper's bugloss is a different plant (an echium).

It is a perennial plant with rather bristly leaves and intense blue flowers, somewhat similar to borage, and is an important food source for bees and butterflies. It is a deep rooting plant and happy in shade under trees.

The root is used as a dye, providing a red colour, and it is possible that the name alkanet came from the Arabic word for henna which was used as a dye for hair and nails, although it is not the same plant.

Culpeper used it and recommended it both internally and as an ointment for green wounds. However, although sometimes used medicinally today, it is <u>not</u> recommended for domestic use.

Aloe Vera
Aloe barbadensis

Aloes are succulent plants, part of the lily family. The leaves are thick, fleshy, and grow in a rosette. They are not hardy in this country, needing a minimum temperature of 5°C (41°F) to survive, and require protection over winter.

It is a plant with an ancient heritage pre-dating the Christian era. In John 19: 39-40, Nicodemus brought a mixture of myrrh and aloes and wrapped the body of Jesus with linen and spices.

In recent times the gel has come to the fore as a cure for skin problems. A leaf broken and applied to a burn will provide a soothing antiseptic cover and bought preparations can ease eczema and similar ills. It is possible to find it prepared for internal use, but this is best taken only after professional advice.

Angelica
Angelica archangelica

A tall biennial which can grow up to 8ft in height, it has a mass of small, yellow flowers which together look like a magic ball. The large, rounded seed heads which follow can be dried (and possibly fixed with hair spray) to make a striking winter decoration.

There is an old legend that the virtues of the plant were revealed to a monk by an angel during a terrible plague and thus it got its name. Along with garlic and sticador or French lavender, it was reputed to be one of the ingredients of Thieves Vinegar – so called because the men who cleared plague ridden houses dosed themselves with this brew and seemed to be immune.

Angelica grows happily as far north as Norway and Lapland and is, therefore, a good plant for colder, less sunny places. To propagate, it is essential the seed is fresh. It is best sown where it is needed as transplanting, except in the seedling stage, is not easy.

A valuable plant with uses far beyond the traditional green, candied cake decoration. When making rhubarb jam, the leaves will add flavour and take away the acidity. The leaf, preferably when young, can be added to salads or as an added flavour to soups or stews. The roots can be dried, grated, and used with flour in a bread mix; they can also be boiled and chopped to make into chutney. Angelica is also an ingredient in the liqueur Chartreuse

Medicinally, the tea would be a mildly stimulating tonic useful in chest infections with a warm taste which can also ease indigestion.

Anise
Pimpinella anisum

A native of Egypt and the Middle East, this is a small annual plant. It will do well in a warm sunny place because it needs the sun to bring it to maturity. The leaves can be added to salad or used as a garnish, but it is the seeds that are the most prized part of the plant. These were an ingredient of Roman spiced cakes and added to curry and other spiced foods.

It is an excellent digestive both warming and comforting to a chilled, unhappy body.

In view of the fact that it takes about 50lb of seed to produce 1lb of anise oil and that the plant can take three or four months to ripen enough to pick, it is not practical to grow it on a commercial scale in this country.

The trade apparently also uses the distilled essence of Star Anise *Illicium anisatum*, a small, Far Eastern tree, to help bulk out the manufacture of aniseed balls and other products.

Anise Hyssop
Agastache anethiodora

A perennial plant of North American origin which looks rather like a tall mint. Indeed, a relation *Agastache ragosa* is called Korean Mint and was known as a remedy in China as far back as the 5th century.

The long, close-knit spikes of purple flowers tend to bloom in full summer and are, therefore, of extra use to bees and butterflies. Since it does not send out runners like a mint, it will make an attractive addition to any flower border.

The anise scented leaves will make a refreshing tea and were used by some American tribes to relieve coughs.

Arnica, Leopard's Bane
Arnica montana

A perennial, low growing plant with yellow, daisy-like flowers. A native of the mountainous regions of Central Europe.

As an instant relief for bruises, the ointment is second to none, although it should not be used where there is damage to the skin.

I have known it to be used in homoeopathic dosage as a support for trauma and to prepare for surgery, dental work, and the like. According to Deni Bown, it is used for heart problems in Germany, for external use only in England, and is ruled unsafe in America.

Balm of Gilead
Cedronella triphylla

A half-hardy, shrubby plant with fragrant leaves and purple flowers. It is a good plant for an unheated conservatory or would grow out of doors in a sunny, sheltered position.

The name *Cedronella* is possibly a reference to the pleasant cedar like scent of the leaves. The dictionary defines 'balm' as 'an aromatic oily resin exuded by various, chiefly tropical, trees and shrubs and used in medicine'. This plant, however, is so named simply because of the perfume which is similar to that obtained from the Eastern trees and used in Olbas Oil to ease catarrh and other problems.

The leaves would add a sharpness to pot-pourri and, according to Deni Bown, can be made into a tea. It has no known therapeutic properties; it is just an attractive plant which gives off its fragrance as you brush past.

Lemon Balm
Melissa officinalis

A vigorous, herbaceous plant which looks rather like mint, but which does not send out runners. It is sometimes called lemon mint or lemon sage. The small, white flowers attract bees and it is a must for anyone who appreciates having something which is undemanding and useful. However, it is a good idea to cut down the flowering stalks as it can self seed readily. Gerard suggests planting near beehives to encourage the bees to return home. The leaves can be rubbed on wooden furniture to give a gloss and fresh scent.

It can be added to stuffing, salads, and so on, and goes well in baked apples. Stuff the fruit with a mixture made up of 2 teaspoons of ground almonds or breadcrumbs, 1 teaspoon of finely chopped balm, 1 teaspoon or more to taste of brown sugar, and a knob of butter. Bake as usual.

A tea of fresh or dried leaves is a notable relaxant, soothing to a digestive upset and, with a small spoonful of honey, will aid sleeplessness which is caused by nervous tension. It is an excellent remedy for children or the elderly and extremely safe.

A spirit of lemon balm combined with lemon peel, nutmeg, and angelica root enjoyed a great reputation under the name of Carmelite Water, being a sovereign remedy for headaches and neuralgia. According to Mrs Grieve it was one of the factors in the longevity of a Prince of Glamorgan, who lived to be 108, and of others who lived to a great age.

Golden lemon balm, with its golden foliage, prefers light shade as it will scorch in direct sun. Variegated lemon balm has green and gold leaves and also enjoys light shade.

Sweet Basil
Ocimum basilicum

Basil is a herb with many different cultivars grown today. The standard one is called Sweet or Neapolitan or Lettuce leaved. It is tender, with sunshine and day length an essential requirement for germination in this country. The winter supermarket supplies will probably be from Spain or Israel. It seems to be one of the 'must have' herbs although 20 or so years ago any herbs except parsley and bay were regarded with suspicion by most people.

Pesto sauce is a mix of olive oil, pine nuts, and basil. Pound basil, pine nuts, and garlic in a mortar. Add grated parmesan cheese or similar, then add olive oil carefully until it is the consistency of cream butter. Elizabeth David suggests using a handful of each ingredient but that is for the individual taste to decide.

The opportunities for use are limitless. Basil is a must with tomatoes, but try it also with pea or lentil soups. Any salad will benefit from a shredded leaf or two.

The Holy basil *Ocimum sanctum* is probably the one reputed to have been brought from India by Alexander the Great. This is a small, aromatic, shrubby plant which is traditionally planted in the courtyards of Indian houses or temples to protect those who cultivated it from misfortune. The Sanskrit and Hindu name is *tulasc* and it is the herb of Vishnu the Protector.

Now being grown successfully in this country, a perennial variety known as African Blue is a more sturdy plant which will survive through the winter if kept on a warm, preferably north facing, window ledge.

Basil Thyme
Acinos arvensis

A low growing, short-lived perennial and originally a wild plant of arable land and grassy areas. It will fill in a gap in a rockery or between paving stones. I have only once seen it growing wild and that was by the concrete base of a dismantled wartime Nissen hut.

The flowers can add colour and flavour to a salad although they are nowhere near as strong as the native wild thyme. Gerard says: 'It taketh away sorrowfulness and maketh a man merry and glad.'

Bearsfoot
Helleborus foetidus

A perennial woodland plant, now rare in the wild, it gives good ground cover in a shrubbery. It has unusual green flowers in early spring.

The Christmas Rose or *Helleborus niger* is also a woodland plant originally found in the wild. The *niger* refers to the black root stock. The white flowers of the Christmas Rose really can flower in the depth of winter and provide a promise of spring when the winter begins to drag on. Both plants were used medicinally in the past, but are poisonous except in homoeopathic doses.

The hellebore family has been developed into a very attractive garden plant with many different coloured flowers, both single and double.

Bergamot
Monarda didyma

A perennial woodland plant of North American origin which is also known as Bee Balm and Oswego Tea. A very attractive plant with scented leaves and clusters of flowers at the top of the stem looking rather like a small red mop. It grows like mint although it is not so rampant and tends to disappear in winter so the position needs marking and preferably covered with leaf mould.

Native Americans valued this plant very highly as a treatment for bronchial complaints, the volatile oil having antiseptic properties.

The leaves will make a tea rather like Earl Grey in flavour, but the oil which is used to enhance the Earl Grey tea comes from a Middle Eastern tree. You can add the leaves to an ordinary black tea and have your own distinctive brew.

You could try marinating a pork chop in a mixture of chopped leaves, oil and seasoning. Leave for an hour then grill and serve with apple rings and cider sauce. The flowers could be added to salad or simply used to add colour to pot-pourri.

There are several different cultivars with pink, white, or purple flowers, all of which are attractive. However, to be successful you need to use the original.

Bay Sweet Laurel
Laurus nobilis

Frequently seen these days as an ornamental shrub, clipped to form a spiral shape or a standard with a ball on top. Given the right conditions it will make a very handsome evergreen tree and you will have the leaves available for culinary use on your doorstep. They are perhaps slightly stronger if dried, but who would want to use them like that if they had fresh leaves at hand? The tree also provides a bonus with very pretty perfumed creamy white flowers.

The *nobilis* part of the name shows in what high regard the plant was held. To be crowned with a laurel wreath was a symbol which was coveted by ancient Greek and Roman leaders. It was also awarded to poets as a symbol both of light and learning with its connection to Apollo the sun god. The French term *baccalaureate* comes also from the crowning with wreaths of laurel berries *bacca laurea* and is now used to symbolise the successful passing of exams.

An ingredient in the 'Bouquet Garni' as advised by Mrs Beeton. This consisted of: 'A sprig of parsley, bay leaf, thyme, and marjoram', although she says they are not indispensable if not easily procured. I think, with the growth in foreign travel and interest in other cuisines, this would not be acceptable today. A bay leaf can be added to soup or stew or any savoury dish, try it with the garlic and herbs when you cook chicken.

It is not normally used medicinally, but it does aid digestion when used as a culinary herb, although Culpeper lists numerous virtues for it.

Bistort
Polygonum bistorta

Also known as Sweet Dock, this is an attractive, easy to grow, perennial native to damp mountain meadows in Europe and Asia. It is also naturalised in North America where it is sometimes called Snakeroot because of the very twisted roots. It has leaves which look rather like dock and spikes of fat, pink flowers.

Tea made from the leaves can be used as a mouthwash for ulcers and to encourage healthy gums. The juice could be effective against heavy bleeding and as a wound healer. The roots contain considerable starch and have been used as a famine herb.

The plant was used in various ways as a spring tonic. A Yorkshire dock pudding championship was held annually with variations based on 2lb bistort leaf, ½lb young nettle tops, and 2 onions boiled with 3 tablespoons of oatmeal, formed into patties and fried in bacon fat. The young leaf could be chopped and added to mashed potato in the same way you would add other green herbs.

In the Lake District, traditional recipes include the first spring cabbage, fresh leaf of bistort, nettle tops, water-cress, newly burst leaves of the soft fruit bushes, mint, Jack-by-the-hedge (Garlic mustard) and a few dandelion leaves and chives or onion. Wash, chop and boil in a bag with barley and oatmeal to thicken. When cooked, turn out, slice, and add a knob of butter and seasoning.

Betony
Stachys officinalis

Once a sovereign remedy of monks giving it its other name of Bishopswort. It was used for treating headaches, especially those caused by an upset stomach or nervous tension. To be avoided if pregnant.

According to *The Physicians of Myddfai*: 'He who will habituate himself to drink the juice will escape the stranguary', an old word for hernia. A Saxon herbal says: 'Betony is good for a man's soul and his body', hence its use to protect against witchcraft. Even earlier, a physician to the Emperor Augustus named Antonius Musa, wrote a treatise praising the plant.

Betony can be found naturalised in meadows with its flower spikes varying in colour from pale pink to magenta, rising from clump forming leaves which are wrinkled and aromatic. The garden plant known as Lamb's Ears is related, but does not have the medicinal qualities.

A Lancashire recipe for a green salve used before 1870 is a handful of balm, sage, southernwood, rosemary, betony, chamomile, lavender, feverfew, red rosebuds and wormwood. Strip from stalks and cut fine, simmer in fresh lard for 2 to 3 hours, and strain. Rub the bruise gently. For an inward bruise, add a nut of salve to hot beer at bedtime.

Borage
Borago officinalis

A sturdy annual with rather wrinkled leaves and bright blue, starry flowers with a black 'eye'. It will self seed freely and the seedlings can be used: chopped into a cottage cheese adding a faint cucumber flavour or added to coleslaw or potato salad. They can be cooked like spinach, but I think they would be better added to another green vegetable to enhance the flavour.

The leaves used to be steeped in wine and since the old saying is: 'Borage gives me courage', it was drunk by Knights before tournaments or a battle. Ladies embroidered the flowers onto scarves to present to their chosen warrior. This practise could be the origin of the borage flowers added to Pimms.

The flowers can be dried carefully and then candied. One recipe is: add 1 cup of water to 1lb caster sugar, bring to the boil, drop in the dry flowers carefully a few at a time and leave in for about a minute. Take out carefully, drain, and leave to cool and dry in a warm place. If you like the flavour, use occasionally as a salad herb.

Used medicinally it will have a tonic action, but as with so many herbs more is <u>not</u> better. Discuss with a herbalist.

Creeping Borage
Borago laxifolia

A perennial, low growing relative of the annual plant. Although the leaves have the same cucumber taste, they are much more prickly. The flowers are also similar, but a pale blue without the black 'eye'. An attractive ground cover plant, but not normally of use otherwise.

Box
Buxus sempervirens

Strictly speaking, box has no place in a herbal, but it has been used clipped into low hedges to surround herb gardens for hundreds of years. Left to itself it will make a small, slow growing tree and there are still one or two places in England where it grows wild.

A decoction of the leaves was believed to prevent premature baldness but it is <u>not</u> recommended for it could have very unpleasant side effects (and probably would not work anyway).

Sprigs and wreathes of box were often laid on graves or carried by mourners at a funeral. It symbolises immortality and perpetuity as do many other evergreen plants.

The wood is a bright, yellowish brown, hard and close grained, and is used for making rulers, precise drawing instruments, and tool handles, as well as being the favoured wood of engravers like Thomas Bewick.

With the interest in gardens and structural plants there are now many varieties available; variegated, golden and with interesting shapes.

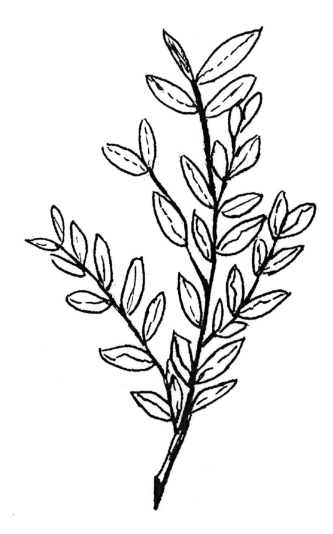

Broom
Cytisus scoparius

An erect shrub with long, stiff, bright green branches which grows on moorland, sea coast, and unused ground. It flowers profusely with yellow, fragrant blooms followed by black seed pods which burst open with a sharp snap. It self seeds readily and will soon take over an unused area.

The Plantagenet kings used Common Broom (*planta genista* in Latin) as an emblem, hence their name.

According to Gerard, King Henry VIII was: 'Wont to drink the distilled water of broom flowers'. The pickled buds were considered a delicacy in the time of the Tudors. The green tips were added to ale to provide the bitterness before hops were used and the tannin in the bark was used to cure leather. The stems were bound and made into brooms hence the common name.

There is evidence of a powerful medicinal effect but it is not one to use domestically.

Dyer's Broom
Genista tinctoria

Also known as Dyer's Greenwood, it is a small shrub related to the broom with a more delicate air. It has yellow flowers which grow in spikes and these give the reason behind its name.

Flemish immigrants in the 14th century introduced a method of turning the yellow dye obtained from the flowers into a green colour. Cloth was dipped first in the yellow and then a second time into the blue of woad. This became known as Kendal Green from the area where it was first developed.

It has been used medicinally, as have most plants through the ages, but has never been an official drug.

Bugle
Ajuga reptans

Another attractive ground cover plant which will grow in damp shady places. It has green leaves and spikes of deep blue flowers. There are now variants of the *reptans* that have bronze or purple leaves and also one with variegated leaves.

It has aromatic and astringent properties and can be used to arrest both internal and external bleeding, but only under professional supervision.

Culpeper says: 'Many times those that give themselves much drinking are troubled with strange fancies, strange sights in the night or voices. These I have known cured by taking only two spoonfuls of the syrup of this herb 2 hours after supper on going to bed.' One wonders if it really worked.

There are varieties of this plant which grow in Africa and Australia which are being investigated as treatment for life threatening diseases.

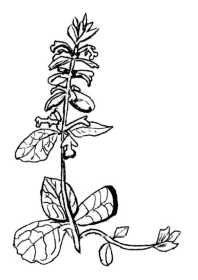

Burdock
Arctium lappa

A tall, perennial herb native to Europe and Asia, but also found in North America. A spectacular wild flower that can reach 3 or 4 feet in height. The purple flowers produce the burrs which all children used to know and are reputed to have been the inspiration for Velcro.

A blood purifying and soothing herb, it has been in use for centuries. Henry III is reputed to have been cured from syphilis thanks to this plant, and it has been used to treat arthritis and skin conditions such as eczema.

The young leaf stems can be stripped of the outer skin (if need be) and either boiled as a vegetable and served with butter or added to a salad, cooled with a vinaigrette dressing or raw.

The root is considered a delicacy in some parts of the world. It is also the part of the plant which is used professionally, but all of it is useful medicinally.

Greater Burnet
Sanguisorba officinalis

An attractive, erect perennial border plant with striking dark red flowers which, according to an old gentleman in our village, were once used to make wine or beer. He told me that 'them old burny knobs' made a wonderful drink. I admit I've never tried it.

The roots have been used in Chinese medicine for more than 2000 years as a wound herb for internal or external healing, but like many remedies it is best left to the professional.

Salad Burnet
Sanguisorba minor

As the Latin name suggests, it is a smaller relation of *Sanguisorba officinalis*. The leaves form an attractive rosette which stays green throughout the year. It is sometimes known as the Fountain Plant from the way it grows with the flower stems rising from the green.

It has a nutty, cucumber flavour so it can be chopped and added to a cottage cheese or to a salad in winter when green is in short supply. If added to a soup or stew, put in at the last minute as it is best when almost raw.

It has similar medicinal properties to the *officinalis* and according to Culpeper it is: 'A most precious herb, the continual use of it preserves the body in health and the spirit in vigour.'

Butterbur
Petasites hybridus

A large leaved plant of damp ground. The flowers, which come first, are on thick stalks with a clustered crown; they are usually pink, but are sometimes white. The thick, almost furry leaves which appear as the flowers decay were used, so it is said, to wrap newly churned butter to help to keep it cool.

Culpeper considered it a sovereign remedy against the plague. The root is the part used; it is made into a tincture for neuralgia and some heart problems.

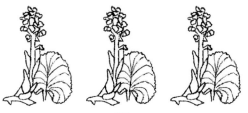

Greater Calamint
Calamintha grandiflora

Also known as Mountain Balm, this is a perennial plant which is aromatic and hardy. It has flowers which are a dark pink and looks rather like catnep in habit although it is also closely related to ground ivy. It is one more plant that is widespread in Europe and was mentioned by both Gerard and Culpeper, but was probably in use well before then. The leaves have a pleasant minty scent and will make a refreshing tea with perhaps some honey added. This can be used as a digestive if needed, but is good just as itself.

Lesser Calamint
Calamintha nepeta

A low growing, ground cover perennial that has small, greyish leaves and pale pink flowers. This plant is also aromatic, but the leaves are not as enticing to the taste. Mrs Grieve says that it is probably stronger and more useful medicinally.

Bladder Campion
Silene vulgaris

A perennial wild flower which used to be common on the headlands of fields and along the roadside. It has a white flower with a kind of round sac or bladder where it joins the stalk, possibly developed through the ages to ensure pollination. It has grey-green leaves which were recommended as a vegetable; the young shoots were boiled and served with butter, or added to a salad, the flavour reputed to be that of green peas.

Red Campion
Silene dioica

A plant which needs two to provide the seed, each being either male or female. Again, a wayside plant, with a white variety as well and many cross pollinations resulting in variations of pink. As far as I can find out, it was not suggested as food although I have no doubt in time of shortage it would do little harm.

The roots can be boiled and will provide a gentle lather but if you have soapwort available that is preferable.

Caraway
Carum carvi

Not a native of Britain, but a biennial with its origins in the Middle East and Asia where it has been cultivated for thousands of years. Used by the Egyptians, mentioned in the Bible, and added to bread for Roman soldiers, it has been a culinary herb of great value.

We tend to think of it as providing the gritty bits in seed cake, one you either like or loathe, but there is much more to it than that. The root can be boiled to add flavour; the young feathery leaves can be chopped and added to a salad; but it is mostly for the seed that it is grown.

As a digestive and a seasoning it has no equal. It enhances roasted onions and most other root vegetables; goes with marrow, spinach, or cabbage for sauerkraut; and can be added to cheese, soups, and stews. In fact, it will go anywhere sweet or savoury if you like the taste. It is the essential oil of caraway that flavours the liqueur Kummel.

An infusion will soothe an upset stomach and it forms an ingredient of the compound tincture Cardamom Aromatica.

Catmint
Nepeta mussinii

A perennial plant with grey, fragrant leaves and spires of blue flowers. It makes an excellent edging plant which is loved by bees. Being a grey leaved plant it is happy in dry, sunny places and will make a cushion of leaf and flowers.

There is no more attractive sight than a moggy asleep in a big plant of catmint. It may be flattened a bit, but will spring back unless the cat has nibbled it; for some felines it is an irresistible treat. One of ours could often be seen, paws in the air, looking somewhat drunk. The leaves retain their scent when dry so can be used in pot-pourri, cat toys, and so on.

Catnep
Nepeta cataria

Also known as catmint, this is a taller, more mint-like perennial plant. This is the one with the medicinal uses. A tea can be made with the leaf, fresh or dried, and it is both warming and refreshing. It is a calming drink and a countryman's remedy for a head cold.

Greater Celandine
Chelidonium majus

A plant of the hedgerow and banks, it is a herbaceous perennial with seed that produces an oil on which ants feed, helping to spread the plant. This yellow flower of the poppy family is not related to the Lesser Celandine although the flower colour is similar.

The most striking property of the plant is the thick, orange sap which exudes from every damaged leaf or stem. This is a traditional remedy for warts and corns, the fresh juice being dabbed directly onto the skin, but do not get it anywhere else because it will stain. This remedy has been in use since before the Roman conquest of Britain. The juice was also used more perilously for clearing cloudiness from the eyes.

The doctrine of signatures suggested its use for liver disorders, the colour of the sap being almost that of bile. A tincture is prepared homoeopathically but apart from the possible use as a cure for warts do <u>not</u> attempt any self medication.

Lesser Celandine
Ranunculus ficaria

A low growing plant with round, shiny leaves and golden, buttercup-like flowers which close up in dull weather. It flowers in the early spring, preferring damp, shady places in woodland and similar sites. The whole plant will disappear as the summer advances, to rest until the day length begins the life cycle again.

The other name for the plant is Pilewort as it has been used since the Middle Ages as a cure for haemorrhoids, either internally as a tincture or as a soothing ointment, which was once made with lard and, more recently, with petroleum jelly.

Centaury
Centaurium erythraea

A meadow and wayside biennial plant. It used to be common but, like many of the less tough, so-called weeds, is now quite hard to find growing wild. The leaves are arranged in pairs up the stem and the pink star-like flowers are in small clusters at the top. The plant is usually no more than 1 foot tall and the flowers are sensitive to light, not opening until the morning is well advanced and closing at dusk, or possibly staying closed on a dull day.

The name comes from the legend that the centaur, Chiron, who was a great healer, cured himself from an injury with this plant. One version says that Hercules accidentally wounded him with an arrow, another that it was damage done by the nine headed Hydra. It does mean, however, that it has been used since ancient days.

Culpeper recommended it as a general tonic and it is used today especially where the digestive system needs support. To be avoided if pregnant.

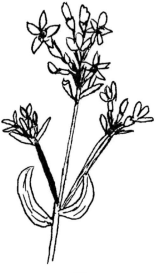

Double Chamomile
Anthemis nobilis 'Flore Pleno'

Used since Saxon times when it was known as *maythen*, a Greek word originally meaning 'earth apples', referring to the wonderful perfume which comes when the plant is brushed or trodden on.

This herb and those related to it are still popular today; even in the days when herbs were a specialist interest, most people would know to use a chamomile rinse for blonde hair to bring out the highlights, even if they did not drink the tea.

The plant is a low growing, spreading perennial that has white pompom flowers in mid to late summer which can be dried for use in winter. They tend to be more bitter than the smell suggests, so honey is a good addition to an infusion. This is a specific, harmless remedy for tension headache, upset stomach and a good tonic for the nervous system in general.

The flowers can also be made into a soothing oil. If not allergic to nuts, almond oil is one of the best to use. Pack a jar with as many flowers as are available, top up with the oil, so they are covered. Keep on a sunny window ledge for about two weeks and then strain and use for any minor skin problems or ear infections.

Dyer's Chamomile
Anthemis tinctoria

A perennial plant of the same family but with yellow daisy-like flowers providing an orange-brown dye.

Roman Chamomile
Anthemis tinctoria

A plant with similar characteristics to Double Chamomile, but with taller flower stems and single, white daisy-like flowers. This is the one which would have been used to dose Peter Rabbit after eating too many of Mr McGregor's lettuces.

This is the original chamomile used for lawns which needed an occasional mow and a roller to keep it level and green. In the latter part of the century a variety was developed which did not flower and so provided easier cultivation.

Lawn Chamomile
Anthemis nobilis 'Treneague'

The variety which has come to the fore recently with Mary Wesley's novel (and television adaptation) *The Camomile Lawn*, not to mention gardening programmes that have mentioned covering a bank of earth with the plant to make a seat.

Lawn Chamomile is not as vigorous as grass or the many weeds such as dandelion which can appear almost from nowhere. Therefore, before planting, it is necessary to make sure the earth is as clean and weed free as possible. The 'little apple' perfume is the same and the small florets will spread through the summer, probably needing one or two replacements for bare patches in spring.

Chaste Tree
Vitex agnus-castus

A small, ornamental, hardwood tree, it appreciates a sunny position as it comes originally from the Mediterranean. According to Mrs Grieve, Greek women used the leaves in the sacred rites of Ceres, named Demeter by the Romans. She was the Earth goddess of cereals: wheat and other grains.

Sometimes called Monks' Pepper, the seeds were ground and used as a condiment. It is a regulator of hormones, hence its common name Chaste Tree, and it is used by professionals to ease some of the discomforts of the menopause and allied problems.

Chervil
Anthriscus cerefolium

One of the many plants which came to Britain with the Romans, it is not as well known as parsley, which is a shame as it is not used enough. A delicate looking annual or biennial plant with lacy leaves and white flowers, it is a relation of Cow Parsley *Anthriscus sylvestris* which is also known as Kek or Queen Anne's Lace.

They both have a warm, slightly aniseed flavour, but the wild variety, although harmless, is much coarser in texture. Do not pick unless you are absolutely certain of identification, as there are similar plants such as hemlock which are poisonous.

Chervil is easy to grow and, sown in the spring and autumn, will provide green throughout the year. It does suffer in long periods of hot sun and does not really like being transplanted so is best sown direct in the garden in a moist, shady spot.

It is one of the ingredients of the 'Fine Herbes' and 'Bouquet Garni', but is at its best when uncooked and added as required. Try it with scrambled egg, potato salad, or just as decoration instead of parsley.

It was a valued medicinal herb in the Middle Ages and is a warming digestive and tonic especially for the brain and memory.

Chicory
Cichorium intybus

Also known as succory, chicory is a perennial plant with a good sized tap root when grown in good earth. In the early stages of growth it looks rather like a dandelion, the rosette of leaves at the base being slightly indented.

The flowers are a beautiful blue and bloom along a tall stem, opening and closing with the daylight hours. These flowers can be used in salads, as can the young leaves; shred a few and combine with lettuce, as they can be quite bitter.

Older leaves can be covered in boiling water and, after 5 minutes, drained and chopped. Add the herbs marjoram, thyme, and parsley and simmer together preferably in a chicken or vegetable stock.

The whole plant is rich in minerals and has been used as a combined food and tonic since Roman times or earlier. The roast and ground roots are added to coffee not as an adulterant, as many believe, but to make it more digestible and a tonic for the liver.

The root can be boiled as a vegetable on its own as one does parsnips or can be combined with cheese and brawn. Parboil the chicory, drain, reserving the liquid to use with added milk and make a cheese sauce. Put diced bacon in an ovenproof dish in layers with the chicory and cover with the sauce, top with breadcrumbs, dot with butter, and cook in a hot oven for about 30 minutes.

To provide leaf in winter, lift the roots, cut off the tops and place in sand or peat under the staging of the greenhouse. This will provide blanched and delicate leaf in winter.

On top of all the human uses, the leaf has been grown as a fodder crop for cattle. My goats always snatched a bite or two on their way past the rows.

Chickweed
Stellaria media

A plant that is more valuable than generally supposed. Rich in copper, it makes an excellent addition to a salad when the leaves are young (it goes stringy later). It can also be made into a soup. Make sure the leaves are well washed and picked over before adding to onion which has been chopped and sautéed in butter. Allow to cook gently for a few minutes before stirring in flour, then add either water or milk, and seasoning to taste. Simmer for 15 minutes then sieve and no one will believe it is not spinach soup.

I have used it in sandwiches when lettuce was scarce and persuaded those who ate it that it was special 'Bench Cress'!

It is a wonderful healer either as a tea to soothe an inflamed stomach or as a poultice for sores and boils. Take a handful of the plant, dip it in boiling water, put on the sore, cover it with a cabbage leaf or something similar, and hold in place with a bandage. Change frequently as the inflammation is drawn out. There are also various proprietary ointments containing chickweed that are available for eczema and other skin problems.

Chives
Allium schoenoprasum

A low growing perennial with rich purple flowers, the plant makes an attractive edging in the summer for the vegetable bed. The only drawback is that they tend to disappear in winter.

Chopped chives with their mild onion flavour can be added to almost any savoury dish either at the cooking stage or as a last minute addition to things like mashed potatoes or coleslaw. It is a good idea to freeze some chopped in ice cubes for winter use in soups. The flowers make a good garnish.

The allium family is vast and ancient with many varieties used for borders, flower arranging, and so on. However, there are several more with culinary uses. Garlic chives *Allium tuberosum* have flat leaves rather like small leeks and heads of white flowers as do Welsh onions (also known as scallions). The Tree onion or Egyptian onion *Allium cepa Proliferum* group is an interesting plant as small onion bulbs grow on the top of the stems and can be used for flavour or pickling.

Onion in all guises is an excellent remedy or preventative for colds and respiratory complaints. Mum's sovereign remedy was a raw onion sandwich. As a child I didn't enjoy it, but it worked.

Clary Sage
Salvia sclarea

A biennial or short lived perennial; this is an attractive, tall plant with broad, greyish, wrinkled leaves and was originally from the Middle East. The flowers have coloured bracts which can be used for decorating a fruit salad or similar sweet. The young leaves can be made into fritters and they were once used as a pot herb or added to an omelette.

The name is a corruption of 'clear eye' for the mucilage from the seeds was used as a wash for sore eyes.

It is also called Muscatel sage from the practise of adding it, with elderflowers, to a Rhine wine. The essential oil is a favourite with aromatherapists for its gentle, soothing, but tonic nature. According to the Institute of Classical Aromatherapy the soothing properties can cause drowsiness and could possibly intensify the effect of drinking alcohol. It is, therefore, best avoided if driving.

Wild Clary
Salvia verbenaca

Also known as Blue Beard, this is a perennial with rosettes of green leaves and blue flower spikes rising to about a foot in height. Both plants have similar uses although the *sclarea* is also used in soap and perfumery.

Cleavers
Galium aparine

A widespread, annual hedgerow plant with hooked bristly leaves and stems that stick to human and animal passers-by to spread the seed and to aid it in climbing through the hedge, hence its other names of Goosegrass or Sticky-willy. A vigorous plant, it is rich in minerals and a good tonic especially for the lymphatic system. A tea made with a tablespoonful of fresh leaf added to a cup of boiling water and allowed to cool, taken three times a day, could act as a cleanser and ease problems like eczema and possibly sore muscles. The burrs, in the past, have been roasted to provide a drink that is reputed to taste rather like coffee.

Red Clover
Trifolium pratense

A good ground cover plant and one which will make a green manure because it fixes nitrogen in the soil. Probably one of the first plants in cultivation. The flowers are used for tea and the young leaf can be added to salad. This is also a grand plant for cleansing the system, relieving problems caused by a build up of toxins. It can be added to a tonic tea with dandelion and nettle to build up a tired metabolism after the winter.

White Clover
Trifolium repens

White Clover has similar properties to the Red, but is not as powerful. If you have a choice, use the *pratense*.

Coltsfoot
Tussilago farfara

A low growing, perennial plant. The small, yellow flowers, rather like dandelions, are the first to show in February; the thick, felty leaves come later. These provide one of the oldest cough medicines known and were so valuable that apothecaries used the flower as their sign.

A tea can be made with a handful of leaves steeped in a pint of boiling water. Add honey to taste and take a cupful up to 3 times a day. If the cough has not eased in a week, visit your doctor.

It is possible to make syrup with layers of leaves and flowers sprinkled with raw sugar. Leave to settle for up to 2 weeks, strain, and take a teaspoonful as needed.

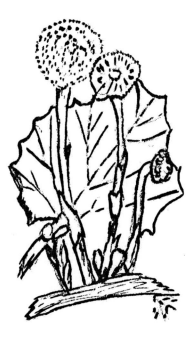

Comfrey
Symphytum officinalis

An ancient herb, this deep rooting perennial of immense healing power is also known as Knitbone. It is so rich that it was one of the wild foods used in survival situations. Some research has been done by force feeding rats with comfrey which then showed signs of liver damage so less is always better – whether it is medicine, alcohol, food or chocolate. As an external remedy for sprains, scar tissue, and so on, it has no equal. There is one important proviso: make sure the wound is clean for it could heal too quickly and fester underneath.

A letter concerning the use of comfrey at a nursing home in Israel states: 'Before using the leaf, she dips it in hot water to get rid of the 'prickly'. She cleans the sore with honey and binds on a leaf, removing it the next day and repeats until the sore is healed.' It is also used for bone injuries in the same way and would be used more but it is restricted by convention.

Added to a bath, an infusion will help with healing ulcers and similar problems. Before research was published into adverse effects if taken internally, I have known it used to relieve a stomach ulcer when drunk as a tea.

It is excellent as a garden fertiliser. The leaves can be used as a mulch or steeped in water with nettles to provide a nourishing liquid with mild insecticide properties.

Coriander
Coriandrum sativum

An eastern Mediterranean annual and an ancient herb mentioned in Exodus 16: 31 – 'And the house of Israel called the name Manna and it was like coriander seed and it was like wafers made with honey.' In view of the fact that it was one of the Hebrew bitter herbs, it is unlikely to be the same plant.

It provides help for the digestion and with the interest in oriental cooking, carrot and coriander soup is popular. Coriander can be used widely; try it with beetroot or celery.

An article in *The Daily Mail* of 24 August 2011 noted: '"Coriander oil could be used to cure a host of infections including food poisoning and MRSA," say researchers. Portuguese scientists tested oil samples against a dozen lethal bacteria, all showed reduced growth and most were killed. The team from the University of Beira are now working on methods of developing as a drug for general use.'

Cotton Lavender
Santolina chamaecyparissus

A small, hardy, aromatic shrub with grey leaves and golden ball-like flowers. The sharply perfumed leaves have been added to pot-pourri, used as a moth repellent, and added to herbal tobacco.

It was once used as a remedy for worms in children. It may ease a bite or sting if a leaf is crushed and rubbed on the affected part. Culpeper suggests adding a decoction to a bath to ease an itch or sore places. Deni Bown says it is not now used medicinally, although research in the 1980s found it to be a valuable anti-inflammatory.

Cowslip
Primula veris

Clusters of yellow flowers rising from rosettes of leaf make the old name St Peter's Keys fit well. A plant of meadows, it has in recent years been seeded alongside some motorways. Although attractive, it is a pity as this limits their availability for use.

The tea is a valuable nerve tonic and is recommended for restlessness and insomnia. Candied or pickled it can be used in puddings and tarts. The young leaf can be added to a salad, but is especially good as a tea or to make wine.

Wild Primrose
Primula vulgaris

Primrose is another well-known perennial plant with its delicate yellow flowers on separate stalks. The *veris* and *vulgaris* have similar properties, but it has been the cowslip which was most used. However, an ointment recipe for sore feet dating from before the First World War, provenance unknown, suggests pounding a handful of *vulgaris* leaves into melted lanolin, to which is added a teaspoonful of thick honey and a few drops thyme oil. This was applied warm to the painful area before covering with cotton socks.

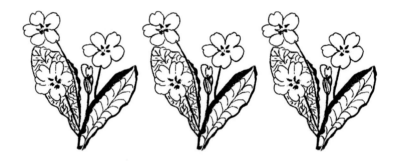

Curry Plant
Helichrysum italicum

A small, attractive, grey leafed shrub with yellow pom-pom flowers rather like cotton lavender, except that the aroma is, as the name suggests, of curry. It is happiest in a dry position and on a sunny day it will scent the air.

You cannot make a curry with it, but you can add small sprigs to rice and so on, giving an extra flavour.

Sweet Cicely
Myrrhis odorata

A perennial herb with lacy, fern-like leaves and frothy white flowers. The whole plant is of use from the roots to the seeds, which can be ground to use as one would a sweet peppercorn. It is an easy plant to cultivate for it will grow on the north side of buildings and is undemanding.

Medicinally it is a digestive, but most people know it for helping to take away the sharpness of fruit, especially rhubarb and apples, thereby needing less sugar.

Daisy
Bellis perennis

A low growing perennial disliked by people who value green lawns. There is an old belief that if you can follow the pink tipped ones they will lead you to faeryland. The young leaf can be eaten in salad; and a salve can be made of pounded leaves mixed with cold cream or similar to ease bad bruising. There is also a homoeopathic remedy used to alleviate swelling as a result of injury. It is still known as Bruisewort in some areas.

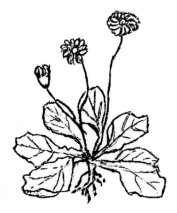

Dandelion
Taraxacum officinale

Another perennial disliked by lawn fanatics, the golden flowers add beauty, but the seed will blow about and spread the plant with its deep roots where it may not be welcome.

Sometimes known as 'Nature's greatest healing aid', it is a diuretic that contributes potassium and is particularly beneficial for high blood pressure problems where there is a build up of fluid. It is also helpful in preventing an accumulation of toxins, which can cause arthritis.

The young leaf can be eaten raw in salad; a good combination is dandelion, chopped chervil, tarragon, and salad burnet with oil and vinegar dressing. Dandelion wine utilises the flowers; the root gently roasted and powdered will make a drink which is caffeine free and a pleasant tasting substitute for coffee.

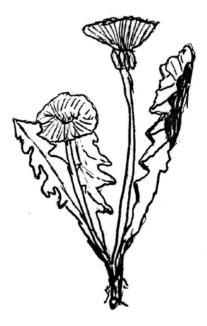

Dill
Anethum graveolens

A half-hardy annual, the name is possibly derived from the Saxon *dillan* ('to lull'), for it is an ingredient of gripe water and soothing to the stomach. An ancient magician's herb ('Dill that hindereth witches of their will') and one of the oldest medicinal plants to be recorded.

The leaf is traditional with salmon and the use of the seed in pickling cucumber and cauliflower is found in recipe books dating from the 17th century.

Elder
Sambucus nigra

A small hedgerow tree with magical associations. The Elder Mother expects respect from those who approach her, as one should have for all living plants and animals as well as humans. There is so much healing power that it is only polite to ask before taking flowers or fruit; and never burn the wood.

The flower will make a soothing ointment that I found effective for nappy rash. They also make a safe remedy for colds; add yarrow and peppermint to the tea if there is fever. My sovereign remedy for warding off a cold is lemon rind and juice, root ginger, elder flowers, and honey to taste. Bring to the boil and allow to steep. Enjoy!

The leaf juice can be used externally for eczema, and the berries make a drink rich in vitamins useful also for coughs and colds. The wine can rival a commercial red any day.

Elecampane, Elfwort
Inula helenium

The plant's specific name, *helenium*, derives from Helen of Troy as the plant is said to have sprung up from where her tears fell. It was sacred to the ancient Celts and also once had the name Elfwort.

This tall, perennial sunflower has been valued for centuries but now seems to have fallen out of favour. It is a good general tonic and also of use for chest complaints. The root used to be candied. A recipe dating from 1577 instructs that the root be sliced and boiled until tender before cooking in sugar syrup. It should then be drained and allowed to dry. Repeat the process two or three times and enjoy as a sweetmeat. I have used dried root to provide a steam inhalation for a hay fever type problem. It was not magic, but it did help a bit.

Evening Primrose
Oenothera biennis

A tall biennial with slightly scented yellow flowers. Of North American origin, it is now naturalised in this country. Earth used as ballast by returning ships is reputed to have shed seed, especially round the docks, and thus this beautiful and useful plant spread and became popular. Following research in the 1980s, oil from the seeds rich in Gamma-linoleic acid is available as a treatment for eczema and arthritis, helping the natural resources of the body.

Fennel
Foeniculum vulgare

A tall, feathery-leafed, handsome perennial with many uses both culinary and medicinal. It is an excellent digestive for rich food and is traditional with some fish. It can, however, be added anywhere to vegetables, salad, or bread.

It used to be called the Meeting Herb as the seeds were given to children in long church services to quiet grumbling tummies. Indeed, it was used in quantity in the Middle Ages both to still hunger pangs and to render suspect food palatable. Medicinally an anti-inflammatory and general tonic, the tea can also be used as a lotion for sore eyes once it has cooled.

'For to make one slender. Take fennel and seethe it in water a very good quantity and wring out, the juice thereof when it is sod [sodden]. And drink it first and last and it shall swage either him or her.' T. Dawson, *The Good Housewives Jewell* 1585

Florence Fennel
Foeniculum vulgare dulce

This is grown for the bulb, the plant being lifted to provide a vegetable.

Feverfew
Tanacetum parthenium

A bushy, aromatic perennial with white daisy-like flowers. It is a traditional remedy for headaches that is now being recognised more widely. An article in *The Independent*, dated 22 July 1988, reports from Nottingham University

Hospital that trials of feverfew have been found to reduce the intensity and frequency of migraine attacks.

Tablets are available, but one or two leaves daily in a sandwich have helped some people. The bread is necessary as a precaution as the leaf is potent and could cause mouth ulcers. Fresh leaf steeped in rubbing alcohol or cider vinegar dabbed on the skin will help to protect from insect bites.

Fig
Ficus carica

A small tree which responds to being root restricted, so it can be espaliered against a wall or even, for some years, grown in a large pot.

It has been known from earliest writings, being mentioned in the Bible. It was also a major article of sustenance for the ancient Greeks. The tree spread from Persia and the Mediterranean countries and was possibly introduced to Britain as early as the Roman period, although for certain from Italy in the Middle Ages.

Small fruits begin to form in late summer to stand over winter, but generally does not survive to grow in spring. However, a new crop appears with the leaves and if you can beat the blackbirds there will be fresh figs by August or September. Large unripe figs can be made into jam.

Many people will associate it with the dreaded Syrup of Figs, which has other things added. It is, however, an important food crop, fresh or dried, and contains many nutrients. Fresh from the tree and beautifully sweet is the best way to enjoy it.

Foxglove
Digitalis purpurea

A woodland plant associated with faery tales, 'fox' being a corruption of 'folk', another name for faeries, the little people who live in the wild. An attractive biennial or sometimes perennial plant, <u>not</u> for self-medication. A Dr William Withering discovered its modern medicinal properties. He was interested in country remedies and experimented with it to help a patient with 'dropsy' caused by a failing heart. He was elected a fellow of the Royal Society for his work. Modern medicine still relies on the drug Digitalin for the treatment of heart problems.

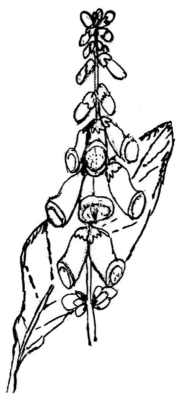

Garlic
Allium sativum

Whether you dislike it or enjoy it, garlic is a plant that cannot be ignored. Valuable in cooking, it is for its medicinal properties that it should be revered. In ancient Egypt it was recorded as being an essential part of the pyramid builder's diet, but before that it was already highly regarded for its therapeutic qualities. A powerful antibiotic, there are trials ongoing for use against new superbugs and also for its apparent ability to lower cholesterol levels and treat high blood pressure.

If you are concerned by the way its odour can linger after eating, try chewing a leaf of parsley.

Elephant Garlic
Allium ampeloprasum

As far as I can find out it is not a hybrid, but was discovered in 1941 in a fertile valley in Oregon, USA. It was in a settlement populated by descendants of settlers from Czechoslovakia and Yugoslavia, who may well have imported it.

Elephant Garlic is not a true garlic but belongs to the onion family, a variant of the species to which leeks belong. It has long, flat leaves like leeks, with strong, tall stems and large, round flower heads of white with a tinge of lilac. It produces a large bulb with four or five cloves the size of shallots which have a mild garlic flavour.

Gingko, Maidenhair Tree
Gingko biloba

An elegant and useful deciduous tree with leaves that turn golden in the autumn. The tree is tolerant of traffic fumes. Both male and female trees are grown, but the female fruits are considered to have an unpleasant smell.

It is one of the oldest living tree species and has been valued by the Chinese for many centuries. The leaves, when processed, may relieve tension and improve blood flow helping to increase alertness, relieve headaches, and so on.

Good King Henry
Chenopodium bonus henricus

Also known as Lincolnshire Spinach, this is a British native wild plant that has been used as a pot herb for centuries. It has the same iron content as spinach and can be cooked in the same way. The flowers should be treated like sprouting broccoli and the young stems like asparagus.

Goat's Rue
Galega officinalis

Also known as French lilac from the very attractive, usually blue, but sometimes white flowers. A herbaceous perennial and well worth adding towards the back of the border.

It was once used to promote the production of milk both in humans and livestock. Culpeper recommends it against fever and pestilence.

Golden Rod
Solidago virgaurea

A perennial, 2ft high, golden beauty that attracts beneficial insects such as lacewings and lady birds.

Culpeper gives it as a sovereign wound herb. It can be used medicinally for urinary problems, but only under professional supervision.

In folk medicine it was thought to bring good luck if grown near the house, possibly because it is a cheerful, undemanding plant.

Ground Ivy
Nepeta glechoma

Also known as Alehoof. This is a creeping plant which is a good source of food for bumble bees. It has been used since Saxon times to add flavour to ale and was in use even after the hop became popular. As a tonic herb, it was sold with others on the streets of London in Elizabethan times. Not to be taken if pregnant.

Hawthorn
Crataegus laevigata

The Nature Conservancy station at Monks Wood did some research on hedgerows in the 1980s and found that original hedges with hawthorn could date back 1000 years and an individual tree could be up to 400 years old. It is a venerable and respected plant with many stories, notably a pre-Christian sacred tree with strong associations with faerie. To sleep under hawthorn trees is to leave oneself open for mischief or enlightenment, depending on the honour you pay them. In Christian mythology it is the plant which supplied the crown of thorns.

Known as Bread and Cheese to children, who nibble the young leaves, the berries make delicious jelly. On a more prosaic level it is a support for an ageing heart and will regulate the circulatory system with no contra-indications known.

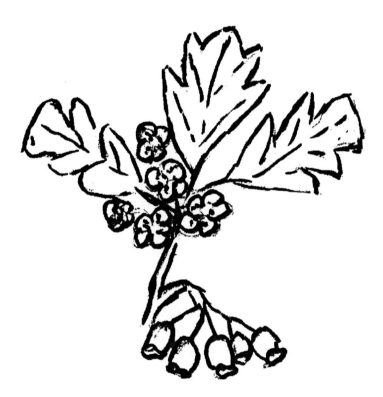

Heartsease
Viola tricolor

A small, wild pansy with colours varying between white, yellow, and purple. Once known as Love in Idleness and used by Oberon to charm Titania (he released the spell with wormwood). Used medicinally, it is a cooling herb which will lower a fever and reduce inflammation.

Sweet Violet
Viola odorata

Mentioned by Shakespeare, this was revered by ancients as a tea, a wine, a sweetmeat (candied), and as a leaf in salads or pottage. With similar virtues as heartsease.

Hemp Agrimony
Eupatorium cannabinum

According to the Reader's Digest *The Wild Flowers of Britain*, Mithradates VI Eupator 120-63BC was a great king and skilled in the use of herbs. It was he who realised the plant's value and gave it its name. It is not a plant for self treatment, although it is valuable in homoeopathy.

It is a tall, handsome perennial, with a mass of tiny, pink flowers which join into a showy head. They prefer damp places and when established will spread along river banks and other waterways.

Herb Robert
Geranium robertianum

An annual or biennial native wild geranium which will self seed readily in any cranny available. The leaves turn an attractive red in autumn, possibly prompting the discovery of the value as a wound herb. Sometimes known as Red Robin, the name probably connects with Puck or Robin Goodfellow, bringing good luck to those who grow and respect it.

The leaves will make a simple mouthwash, which can be of use in treating sore gums, bearing in mind that more is <u>not</u> better. Steep a leaf or two in boiling water and allow to cool before use. This can be strengthened if necessary, but start cautiously.

Holly
Ilex aquifolium

The most important of English evergreens, with sturdy glossy leaves; the ruler of the winter months, as the oak rules in summer. A plant of good omen for it seems invulnerable. I have seen one regenerate over the years from an apparently dead stump into a small but healthy tree. The wood is valuable for marquetry and chessmen and can make an elegant walking stick.

The Bach flower remedies include holly and it can be of medicinal use, but only by professionals. The berries are a powerful emetic.

Holy Thistle
Carduus benedictus

An annual herb with yellow flowers and prickly leaves. It is called 'blessed' for it was considered a cure for all fevers, especially the plague. The young leaf can be eaten and the flower buds treated as globe artichokes, or dried for flower arrangements.

Milk Thistle
Silybum marianum

A tall, striking plant with large, purple flowers and dark green leaves marbled with white; one that can also be used for food or medicine. The young leaf is good in salad, older leaves or the root can be boiled. The plant has recently found popular favour as a liver tonic, a cleanser of toxins from the system, and tablets can now be bought for this purpose.

Hollyhock
Althea rosea

A tall biennial or perennial plant introduced in the 17th century. It was once used as a pot herb, but it is not very tasty. It is a traditional cottage garden plant and possibly the 'Pretty maids all in a row' referred to in the nursery rhyme.

Marsh Mallow
Althea officinalis

A wild relation of the hollyhock, with properties beyond compare. The young leaf can be eaten in salad; the root has unique soothing and lubricating powers. This can provide a protective lining to the gut, helping with problems that range from simple indigestion to acute gastritis. It enables the body to relax and thus aid the healing process. An ancient herb whose pollen was discovered in a cave burial which dated back 60,000 years according to Barbara Griggs.

The sweet is no longer made from the powdered root and sugar, but is now produced with starch and gelatine. It was once seen growing wild in Galloway, but the lane was widened and it disappeared.

There is a tradition that, before being subjected to the ordeal of holding a red hot iron, a person who coated their hands with mallow blended with egg white would be protected.

A recipe of 1723 suggests peeling and chopping the stalks which, when boiled and seasoned with salt and buttered, could pass as 'March Pea'. I admit I have never tried it.

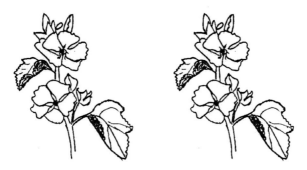

Musk Mallow *Malva moschata*
Wild Mallow *Malva sylvestris*

These are both similar in habit and properties, but are of lesser value than the *officinalis*.

67

Horseradish
Armoracia rusticana

To quote a magazine article by G J Binding: 'An ancient herb full of goodness possibly brought by Romans, the leaf used to soothe aching feet.' Rich in vitamin C and containing mustard oil, which has a disinfectant action, it provides a warming effect with increased blood flow to the tissues thus increasing healing power. The root makes a sauce for rich food, as it is an aid to digestion. Eaten regularly it builds up the immune system. Inhaling fumes from grated root can help to clear sinus congestion. To get a good root you need earth which is fairly stone free, but it will grow anywhere. The young leaves will add piquancy to a dull sandwich.

Houseleek
Sempervivum tectorum

A small, succulent rosette of leaf with pink flowers on short spikes. It is a plant associated with Jupiter and Thor thus protecting the roof on which it is growing from lighting strikes. The juicy leaf is soothing for burns, chapped skin, insect bites, and similar problems.

Hop
Humulus lupulus

A hedgerow climber, it has been widely grown, originally to use as a vegetable. The shoots can be treated like asparagus or chopped into a soup (it makes an excellent addition to green pea). It relaxes smooth muscles, so it is good for tension, upset stomachs, and is traditional for insomnia. Hop pillows have been in use for centuries. If you are making one, try adding lavender or lime flowers. Warning: hops must <u>not</u> be used in cases of depression.

If you are a beer drinker, look for real ale brews as these are less likely to produce a bad head the morning after. Try hop wine it is delicious.

Horehound
Marrubium vulgare

With grey leaves and small white flowers, it is found in dry, waste places. A famed remedy for coughs, the candy was available until recently. A few leaves crushed with honey will help to ward off a cold. If you wish to produce your own candy, make an infusion of a handful of the herb boiled in half a pint of water, strain, and add up to 2 pounds of sugar. Boil until it sets when dropped in cold water, put in a greased tin, and cut when cold.

Hyssop
Hyssopus officinalis

A small, evergreen shrub usually with blue flowers, although they are sometimes pink or white. Bees love it!

It has been used since ancient times to cleanse and purify (it is mentioned in the Bible although this is not necessarily the plant we know today); as a strewing herb to prevent the spread of disease; as a poultice with sugar for cuts when there is a risk of tetanus; and in stuffings or sauces. The flowers or young leaf can be used in salad. A valuable herb, but best <u>not</u> used if pregnant.

Jasmine
Jasminum officinale

A climbing plant with white, scented flowers, it is widely grown for use in the perfume industry. It is hardy and can be long lived; I know of one which is probably 50 years old and flowers every summer.

The essential oil is expensive as extraction is a complex process, but for nervous tension and allied problems it is excellent. Jasmine tea is a lightly scented, usually green tea which has been exposed to the flowers for some weeks.

Juniper
Juniperus communis

An evergreen, aromatic shrub or small tree with male and female plants; both are needed if you want the berries. They are one of the essential ingredients of gin and give it its name (it is derived from either the French *genièvre* or the Dutch *jenever*, which both mean 'juniper').

The branches were used as a disinfectant strewing herb or burned to sweeten the air. As a healing herb, it has a generally cleansing effect, relieving rheumatism and fluid retention. Use with caution and <u>never</u> if you have kidney disease or are pregnant.

Lavender
Lavandula angustifolia

One of the best known herbs, it is a native of the Mediterranean. It was probably brought by the Romans who valued it as a bath herb – for its antiseptic qualities as well as its fragrance.

The plant has so many useful qualities it is hard to list them all. The essential oil is one of the few that can be put directly on the skin instead of needing to be mixed with a carrier oil. Use directly on insect bites or diluted for minor burns. The infusion will ease a headache and provide relaxation for nervous tension.

The leaf can be used in salads or added to a casserole and, of course, the flowers can be dried and put into lavender bags for sleep pillows, the wardrobe as moth repellent, or added to pot-pourri.

A large number of different cultivars are now available. Some varying in flower colour, such as Kew Red *Lavandula stoechas*, the white *Lavandula stoechas* 'Snowman', and so on; some which grow to different heights and others that are less hardy.

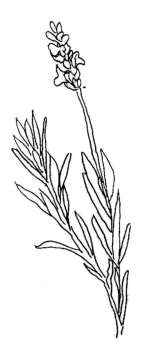

Lemon Grass
Cymbopogon citratus

A tender grass that needs a minimum temperature of 45°F (7°C). It is a useful plant, rich in minerals, used in cooking but also commercially for perfume, soap, and so on.

The leaf, when infused for tea, is a mild digestive. The thick white base of the stems can be chopped and used in cooking.

Lemon Verbena
Lippia citriodora

An attractive shrub, although it can grow to be a small tree in its native home of South America. It is mostly hardy, but needs a sheltered place or some protection in hard frosts.

It has strongly lemon scented leaves and pale lavender spires of flowers. The leaves dry well so that you can make the pleasant relaxing tea throughout the year, or use it when needing a lemon flavour in cooking.

It was once used extensively in perfumery and will certainly add a zing to a pot-pourri.

Linseed
Linum usitissimum

Also known as flax, it is an annual of great antiquity grown as a field crop. Seeds have been found in Egyptian tombs. The stem fibres produce the raw material for linen and the blue flowers set a smooth brown seed which is used in medicines to provide soothing lubrication. The seed can be ground to add to flour for baking (2 tablespoons to 1lb of flour will be enough) or soaked and added to breakfast cereal for some extra goodness.

Lily of the Valley
Convallaria majalis

A perennial once wild in woodlands, with beautiful, delicate, fragrant, white bell shaped flowers. A medicinal herb whose use can be traced back to the 2nd century AD. It is, however, an extremely potent cardiac tonic and must only be prescribed by professionals. The fruit is toxic if eaten.

Lovage
Levisticum officinale

A tall perennial with flat heads of yellow flowers that produce flavoursome seeds. One more herb introduced by the Romans and grown for both culinary and medicinal use. It has a pungent, peppery taste of celery, but is stronger, so that it is best used with discretion. It goes well with lentils and haricots or added to a salad. The young shoots can be blanched and eaten as a vegetable; the seeds can be added to bread or biscuits. A tea may ease colicky pains for it has warming properties and it was once used to help kidney problems. It does not seem to be in the official drug list.

Pot Marigold
Calendula officinalis

An annual; sometimes perennial if it is deadheaded. Once thought of as gaudy with its orange daisy-like flower, it is now recognised as valuable. There has been a proliferation of cosmetics, soothing creams, and so on that contain calendula. The petals have been used to colour cheese and butter, dried to flavour broth and pottages in winter, and made into a tea as an anti-inflammatory remedy. The main virtue, however, is for problems of the skin such as eczema and as a cream for sunburn and slow healing wounds such as leg ulcers.

Wild Marjoram, Joy of the Mountain
Oregano vulgare

A perennial plant, this is the oldest variety of oregano. There are now many different cultivars, some with golden foliage, which are more attractive than culinary. One of the best flavours comes from sweet marjoram, a half hardy perennial usually grown as an annual. There is also a compact marjoram which is a neat, late flowering kind. This helps to extend the season for the many bees and butterflies that rely on the pink and purple flowers of the oregano family.

The herb is much used in Mediterranean type dishes and has properties which make it an aid to digestion, especially of rich foods. The dried herb produced commercially is a blend of various related plants giving it a stronger flavour than the simple leaves.

It was once used as a strewing herb as well as being placed in bags, much as lavender, to keep clothes and their closets fresh.

Meadowsweet
Filipendula ulmaria

Known as Queen of the Meadow although this may originally have referred to mead as it was used to flavour drinks. One of the sacred Druid herbs and a valuable plant, with its frothy, sweet smelling flowers it was also used as a strewing herb. The plant contains salicylic acid, the active ingredient of aspirin, and tea from the flowers can be used instead for similar problems requiring the drug. Dried, they will scent a drawer as does lavender. If cooked with fruit, it lessens the need for sugar. It can also be made into wine.

Mint
Mentha...

There are many varieties of mint, including:

Peppermint – *Mentha piperita*
Which really needs no introduction.

Spearmint – *Mentha spicata*
The original garden mint with its pointed leaf.

Applemint – *Mentha rotundifolia*
This has a round leaf with fruity overtones.

Pennyroyal – *Mentha pulegium*
A creeping plant once used to flavour black pudding and reputed to discourage ants.

All mints have digestive qualities and peppermint is good for chills with its warm feel. It makes a soothing drink.

An old Yorkshire recipe uses chopped mint with dried fruit and brown sugar as a filling for a turnover instead of apple. Mint sauce made with vinegar and brown sugar is a traditional accompaniment to a dish of lamb. Add a sprig to green tea. If you like mint, experiment!

It is possible to buy bags of chamomile and peppermint. This is handy to have available for an upset stomach and the like, but it is much nicer to mix your own and be able to vary the quantities according to need.

Mugwort
Artemisia vulgaris

A widespread perennial wild plant with aromatic leaves and minute yellow flowers. It is a bitter herb which can be added to stuffing for rich meat or as a flavour for ale. It has an ancient background and is known as a Druid herb and a woman's herb, but is not for use if pregnant.

It is said that Roman soldiers put the leaf in their sandals to ease sore feet. It was still recommended in 1656, but this time to ease a footman; not, I think a domestic servant, but one who accompanied travellers.

Wormwood
Artemisia absinthium

A perennial bitter herb, the leaf more grey than mugwort. Used as a strewing herb. The absinthe extracted from the root, made into a drink, can be addictive and deadly. The plant is a good addition to the back of a border, growing to about 3 feet in height with the slightly silky looking leaves providing a good background for more brightly coloured flowers.

Southernwood
Artemisia abrotanum

Also called Old Man, it is a shrubby, feathery-leafed plant with a delightful, sharp, lemony scent, which added to a bath, will cheer and refresh. Sprigs combined with rue were used in court proceedings to protect the judges from fevers. All the artemisias have similar properties to aid digestion, colic, and so on, as well as easing pre-menstrual symptoms. Never to be used if pregnant. Always remember that more is not better.

Mullein
Verbascum thapsus

A tall, biennial with spikes of yellow flowers and thick felty leaves. Also known as Aaron's Rod from its habit and Candlewick Plant because stems were dipped in tallow and used as torches. The flowers are an excellent soother for the chest; a decoction of leaf can be used for mumps and swollen glands and, perhaps with elderflower added, would ease a fever.

Even when losing their first bloom, they are still an attractive plant. It is a host of the Mullein Moth. The moth itself is small and undistinguished, but the caterpillar is wonderfully striped and although it reduces the leaves of the plant to tatters, it is well worth it.

Myrtle
Myrtus communis

A shrub which is normally hardy if happy in its location. Originally from Southern Europe and Asia, it will not grow in a damper, sunless position. A lovely and useful plant with an ancient history, sacred to Venus, the goddess of love and immortality. The white flowers are symbolic of good fortune and peace. Once used in wedding bouquets, notably that of Queen Victoria which brought her not happiness, but the promised prosperity and ripe old age.

Both leaves and berries are of use. The leaves will make a pleasant drink or can be used to add flavour to a meat dish. The small, black berries are reputed to have been served as a digestive at Roman orgies, but are a pleasant nibble at any time. Dried and ground they provide a spice, and the distilled oil from the plant is used in perfumery.

Nasturtium
Tropaeolum majus

An attractive and useful plant, grown as an annual in this country, although in its native South America it is a perennial. It will survive in a conservatory or a heated greenhouse, making a cheerful, colourful hanging basket.

The round leaves and bright flowers can be added to salad or used to sharpen up a dull cream cheese. The seeds are a substitute for capers. A recipe of 1736 says to put the seed in cold salt water for 3 days and then make a pickle of white wine, shallot, horseradish, pepper, salt, cloves, mace, and nutmeg. Put in the seeds and cover.

All parts are of value medicinally having an antibiotic action. According to a book published in Czechoslovakia, this is an unstable reaction so that it is of no interest commercially but valuable in the home.

Nettle
Urtica dioica

A plant that everyone knows, it is reputed to have come with the Romans, who beat themselves with bundles of it to increase blood flow and ease rheumatic pains.

Nettles have been used to make cloth. According to the Reader's Digest *The Wild Flowers of Britain*, a Bronze Age man was found wrapped in a cloth woven of nettle fibre. The tough yellow roots can also be used, twisted to make a sturdy rope.

More valuable, however, is its immense goodness. It is a whole body nutrient. Supremely non-toxic, it can be eaten as a vegetable when young. Cook like spinach with minimal water and a knob of butter, perhaps adding a grate of nutmeg before serving. Dried or fresh it makes a tea that is a tonic rejuvenator. It also makes an excellent beer with many recipes available, although I admit I have never tried it.

Parsley
Petroselinum crispum

A biennial native of the Mediterranean this is often used as decoration, which is an insult to its nutritional qualities. An aid to digestion, it is rich in iron and vitamin C and for a vegetarian or vegan, a daily ration of fresh picked leaf is ideal. It can also be used to ease rheumatic problems and a leaf chewed should purify a 'garlic breath'. Add it to cream cheese, coleslaw, soup, in fact anywhere it will intensify flavour and be good for you as well.

There is a French or Flat-leaved parsley that is supposed to be stronger in flavour. Hamburg or Root parsley provides a root similar in looks to a parsnip that can be added to soups and stews or grated into salad.

Plantain
Plantago lanceolate

Ribwort, also sometimes known by the Saxon name of Waybread, is a plant found in meadows and along grass verges, although it is not one that says: 'Look at me.' The varieties are so widespread that in some places it is known as White Man's Footprint.

It is an astringent herb that promotes healing as well as being a major wound herb. According to Barbara Griggs, an American herbalist named Dr Christopher, who founded a school of natural healing, used poultices of plantain leaves on infected cuts, reinforced with a tea made of the leaves and, apparently, had much success with the treatment. The crushed leaf can also be used on bites and stings and the tea will ease chest infections and catarrh.

Purslane
Portulaca oleracea

An annual herb with yellow flowers and many small black seeds. The leaf is crunchy and slightly salty and was much used in salad in Elizabethan times. It was so valued that it was pickled and preserved for use in winter. Recent research has found it a rich source of Omega 3 fatty acids.

Purple Coneflower
Echinacea purpurea

An attractive, herbaceous perennial from North America, this is a fairly recent addition to the list of medicinal herbs. Trials into its efficacy were held in Germany in the 1930s. Later it was hailed as a cure-all and a stimulant for the immune system. After considerable over use, with tablets easily available, things have settled down to a valuable remedy used with care.

In addition to its medicinal qualities, there is every reason to include it or one of the variously coloured cultivars in the flower garden.

Rhubarb
Rheum rhaponticum

This variety is the traditional garden plant which was developed in the 19th century from the original medicinal plants. The kitchen garden rhubarb has long pink stems which are the edible part and delicious cooked with angelica or sweet cicely, as this helps to calm the acidity of the plant so you can cut down on the amount of sugar you use. The leaf is harmful if eaten. However, if steeped in the water butt, it will provide a mild insecticide.

Chinese Rhubarb
Rheum palmatum

The Turkey or Chinese rhubarb is the principal plant used in medicine. The rhizome is dried and ground to provide a healing and laxative effect. I believe it was the main ingredient of a dreaded medicine of my youth known as Gregory Powder, developed by a Scottish Physician who practised in the early 19th century.

Rocket
Eruca sativa

According to Eleanor Sinclair Rhode, the eating of lettuce without rocket or purslane was forbidden by the Greek physician Galen. A popular plant of the brassica family with pungent leaves, it adds bite to a salad. Although an annual, it is easy to grow to provide a succession.

Wild Rocket
Eruca vesicaria

A long lived perennial with a good flavour. A customer bemoaning the loss of her plant in the bitter winter of 2011, added: 'However, I had had it for nine years!'

Dog Rose
Rosa canina

The true wild rose. The root of the dog rose was used in ancient times to treat infected dog or wolf bites, giving one reason for its common name. Another possibility is that 'dog' is a corruption of 'dag' or 'dagger', an allusion to the thorns.

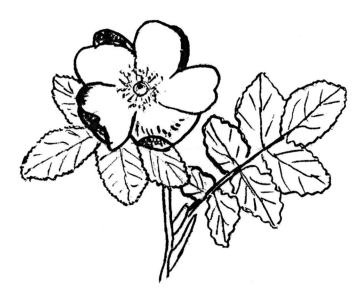

Sweet Briar
Rosa rubiginosa

Walk past the plant after a shower of rain and the scented leaves will refresh the senses, although the leaf, if touched, does not seem to be perfumed. The flowers and hips are similar to the other wild roses. Sweet briar hips were puréed and sieved, then made into a sauce with honey which was served to Queen Victoria at Balmoral and known as Sauce Eglantine.

Hedging Rose
Rosa rugosa

Originally from Japan, this will flower in succession from May to October. Birds love the large, fleshy hips which are a rich source of vitamin C. During the Second World War rose hips were made into a syrup to replace unobtainable oranges. The fruits of any variety will make an excellent jelly and the petals have been used since time began to make rose water for both culinary and cosmetic use.

Apothecary's Rose, Red Rose of Lancaster
Rosa gallica

An ancient and beautiful shrub. Richly perfumed, the plant which the housewife of the Middle Ages would insist on having in her herb garden to use for flavouring, soothing, pot-pourri, and so on.

There is also a striped variety, *Rosa gallica* 'Versicolor', with very pretty and delicate petals, although it does have a tendency to revert to plain colours.

Rosemary
Rosmarinus officinalis

A shrubby native of warm seacoasts brought to Britain by the Romans or even before as an essential culinary ingredient, now traditional with lamb. Ophelia chose rosemary for remembrance. As a symbol of love and loyalty it was given both at weddings and funerals.

The burning of branches was recommended as a precaution to fumigate a sick room, as well as to prevent the plague from spreading into one's home.

It has a sharp, refreshing scent and the essential oil on a tissue clears the head and sharpens the brain – useful for exams or for anyone engaged in intellectual work. A tea made from young tips will have a tonic effect and aid problems of a nervous origin. An old book says that placed under the pillow it will keep away bad dreams, but the sleeper must be without sin for it is a holy tree.

There are now many different cultivars with varied coloured flowers and habit. Sea Level, for example, is a trailing plant with deep blue flowers; Miss Jessup's Upright, is an old and sturdy variety. I like to think of this eminent gardener striding across her land and passing on her character to the plant.

Rowan
Sorbus aucuparia

The Mountain Ash. A long lived, small tree linked to the Celtic ogham, it is believed to be magical, connected with faerie, and able to protect against sorcery. The flowers have a rather unpleasant smell, but the berries hang in bright orange-red bunches and are edible. Each year I hope I will make some sharp tasting jelly, but each year the birds clear the tree before they are really ripe!

The berries have an astringent value and a tea would possibly ease a sore throat or tonsillitis. A few berries should be crushed into boiling water which is then strained before adding honey. This will do no harm and may help.

Rue
Ruta graveolens

A small, evergreen shrub with grey-green pungent leaves, yellow flowers, and a reputation for being dangerous. The action of the sap on skin when combined with sunlight can raise blisters. A sprig worn in the hat will help keep flies away, but tucked under a watch strap, as one lady did, is a recipe for disaster (and it was). A derivative of one of its chemical constituents, coumarin, gives off fluorescence in ultra violet light and according to a 1983 'Herbal Review' this could be the repelling factor.

Perhaps because it is a bitter herb with an association with regret, as in 'rue the day', it was also known as Herb of Grace by Shakespeare, among others. It was used as a strewing herb in the courts; was one of the ingredients of Thieves Vinegar; and was placed in nosegays with other herbs to protect from the plague.

Alison Uttley, when writing of her childhood in Derbyshire, says they were regularly dosed with it, but does not say what benefit it had. It was reputed to have been used as an eyewash by Michael Angelo when painting the Sistine chapel.

The virtues of rue are many and various, not least as an attractive plant for poor dry soil; however it is a herb to treat with the utmost caution. As always, if in doubt consult a professional.

Sage
Salvia officinalis

A potent shrub with various coloured, especially a purple variety, *Salvia purpurascens*; a golden one, *Salvia Icterina*; and one with variegation, *Salvia tricolor*. There is also a narrow leaved plant known as Spanish sage, *Salvia lavandulifolia*, which has an affinity with lavender aroma. All of these have medicinal value, although the *tricolor* is less vigorous and best treated as an ornamental.

The name comes from the Latin for salvation and it is worth more consideration than as stuffing, although this makes use of the digestive qualities. Sage and onion is traditional for the richer poultry and for pork, but it is also added to cheese, notably Sage Derby. Added to toothpaste, it is reputed to whiten teeth and protect the gums. It can also be used as a gargle or mouthwash for sore throats. Add 1oz of sage to 1pt of water with a dash of cider vinegar, simmer for 5 minutes, then cool and strain. Use frequently.

The Chinese valued sage so highly as an aid to longevity, they were prepared to exchange 3lb tea for 1lb dried sage.

It is used in homoeopathic doses for sweats, especially those of the menopause, and as a tonic for older people. Use with discretion – more is not better. Do not use if pregnant.

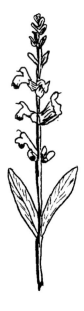

Winter Savory
Satureja montana

An aromatic, low growing shrub with pale purple flowers beloved by bees. Known as the bean herb it discourages flatulence, being rich in volatile oils. There is also a creeping variety, a prostrate plant with white flowers which come late in the season.

Summer Savory
Satureja hortensis

This variety is an annual. Used in quantity by the Romans and mentioned by Shakespeare, it tastes like a peppery thyme. I add it to the garlic when I cook lamb. It goes well with lentils, pea soup, or in stuffing for marrow.

St John's Wort
Hypericum perforatum

A perennial plant with bright yellow flowers, it used to be dried and hung over the doorway to protect from evil spirits. Oil infused with the flowers turns red. Known as Crusader's Oil, it has a reputation for healing nerve tissue, useful after sword fights, but also in today's world for alleviating the pain of neuralgia. There has been an increase in its use as an alleviation for nervous depression, but this should only be taken under supervision for it may react with other medication. For some people it may cause a reaction to sunlight when taken internally therefore, as always, consult a professional.

Soapwort
Saponaria officinalis

Also known as Bouncing Bet, this is a perennial with clusters of pink flowers, the name giving a clue as to its use. The whole plant, but especially the root, produces a gentle lather which can be used as a shampoo or to wash fine fabrics.

For a shampoo, crush half an ounce of soapwort root and wash well. Put it in a bowl and cover with 2pts of boiling water. Allow to steep for an hour then strain. This should be enough for 2 or 3 washes. The addition of a sprig of rosemary or lavender for dark hair or chamomile flowers for fair hair would make it sweet smelling.

Some years ago, tapestries at Burghley House in Stamford were cleaned with Soapwort. It has been used medicinally but is not recommended.

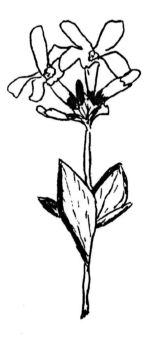

Skirret
Sium sisarum

A garden vegetable known in England since the time of Henry VIII. A perennial plant rather like parsnip, it can be boiled and served with butter – a pleasant addition to the meal.

It is not now used medicinally, but was considered to be restorative and helpful in chest complaints.

Smallage
Apium graveolens

A biennial wild celery, it has a strong smell and is dismissed generally as inedible. However, Richard Mabey suggests using the dried leaves as flavouring and maybe a small number of chopped stems or seed.

It can be an ingredient of medicines for arthritis, as the cultivated variety of celery is reputed to be.

Garden Sorrel
Rumex acetosa

A perennial with leaves like spinach. It has a sharp taste known to children as Sourgrass. Its leaves are used to make sorrel soup; if a chopped potato is cooked with the leaves it will be little milder. The leaves can be added to salads, omelettes, and made into a sauce for fish. Sorrel is rich in oxalic acid and valuable in counteracting the effect of rich food. It is not good for people with gout or other rheumatic problems.

Buckler Sorrel
Rumex scutatus

A perennial plant with similar properties to the Garden sorrel, but with a milder flavour. The leaves are small and shield shaped, mainly used in salads and omelettes. This is also not for people with rheumatic problems.

Tansy
Tanacetum vulgare

A perennial, aromatic herb resembling a sheaf of green feathers topped by dense clusters of golden daisies. A strewing herb, it will dry well and keep its colour. The sharp scent will discourage moths and other unwanted insects. It was once made into puddings as a spring tonic or as a substitute for mint. In our more delicate age there are warnings of toxicity if taken internally.

French Tarragon
Artemisia dracunculus

A perennial culinary herb with insignificant flowers, grown from cuttings. If you are offered seed, it will almost certainly be Russian tarragon – a larger, inferior plant. It is warming and traditional with chicken, but try it elsewhere such as in tomato soup. Leaves steeped in oil or vinegar will add flavour in the winter when the plant is dormant. According to E. S. Rhode, it was first grown here in Tudor times but only in the Royal Gardens.

Thyme
Thymus vulgaris

A small shrub loved by bees and faeries, a symbol of courage, and a plant to refresh the spirit. There are now a multitude of cultivars in various colours and fragrances. They are all useable but not all are enjoyable.

It is an essential ingredient of stuffing, but has many other properties. One of the finest and safest antiseptics, a dilution of Glycerine of Thymol was an essential for a sore throat and it is also used in toothpaste. A mix of 10 drops each of thyme and lemon essential oil diluted in a spray bottle will act as a quick disinfectant in the kitchen or bathroom. One of the earliest medicinal plants used by Egyptians in embalming. Known to Hippocrates and Pedanius Dioscorides, it was used to combat infectious diseases.

The essential oil is powerful and should only be used well diluted in a carrier oil. It should <u>not</u> be used if pregnant.

Valerian
Valeriana officinalis

A perennial with much divided foliage and clusters of small pink flowers rising from deep green leaves. Once used as a pot herb, but now as a nerve remedy, it provides one of the best herbal sedatives and was grown in all monastery gardens for its healing qualities. It can be used for any condition where the nervous system is under stress, as in indigestion, insomnia, or even to ease trauma caused by warfare. It is not a pain reliever and should be used with caution for it would enhance the effect of other allopathic medication. If used long term it can become addictive.

The smell of the roots is attractive to both cats and rats but not to most humans. Perhaps the Pied Piper carried valerian root to enchant the rats.

Red Valerian
Centranthus rubra

This has an attractive red flower and is a plant that will grow almost anywhere. It is not related to *Valeriana officinalis* and has no medicinal qualities. However, the young leaves can be used as greens or as a salad as they are, according to Richard Mabey, in France and Italy.

Vervain
Verbena officinalis

Another plant with insignificant, pale pink flowers on long slender stems. It is hardy and not fussy about where it grows, was once a common wayside plant, and now a great addition to the border. Also known as Enchanter's Herb, it was sacred to many cultures including the Celts and their Druids. A herb 'beneficial in all the ills of man (or woman)' and a magical protector as long as you remember to add a prayer of thanks when lifting it.

For fevers and nervous disorders, it was also once used to treat the plague. As a tea it can be used to inspire and aid intuition. It can also be used as a dental remedy for sore gums. In Chinese medicine it is used to treat malaria for its action is said to resemble quinine.

Weld, Dyer's Rocket
Reseda luteola

Related to Wild Mignonette *Resedua lutea*, this is a tall biennial and an impressive plant with a rosette of crinkled leaves and a spike of tiny yellow flowers which move round and follow the sun during the day.

An ancient dye plant yielding a brilliant yellow dye used mainly in the mediaeval wool industry. However, according to the Reader's Digest, it has been around since the Stone Age.

Woad
Isatis tinctoria

A biennial or short lived perennial with tall yellow flowers followed by dangling black seedpods that will add to a flower arrangement if dried. The blue dye, which was used by ancient Celts to paint their bodies, was extracted from the fermented leaf, a very smelly process according to Mrs Grieve. To satisfy the woollen trade it was once grown commercially in Lincolnshire.

A similar plant has been used in China since 1590 and Deni Bown mentions recent research showing anti-viral effects.

Sweet Woodruff
Galium odoratum

With its small white flowers it makes a good ground cover plant in shade. Once a strewing herb, it was used mainly in churches. As it dries, it smells of new mown hay and is a good moth deterrent. Added to a white wine it is a pleasant tonic. Taken as a tea it should calm nervous tension and provide a harmless tranquillizer for headaches and sleepless nights.

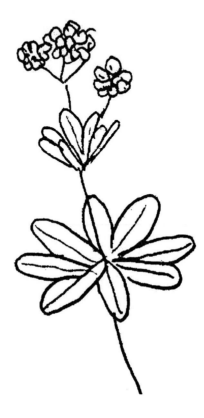

Squinancy
Phuopsis stylosa

Related to sweet woodruff, it is similar in habit, but with pink flowers that appear from June till late October. Very attractive to butterflies and bees. The name derives from its reputed efficacy as a gargle for quinsy, although it is not now used, sage being a better treatment.

Yarrow
Achillea millefolium

The wild grassland variety in a large family of achillea. A perennial with feathery pungent foliage and heads of small, usually white flowers clustered together to form a flat head. Native to the British Isles, it has been used through the ages, notably by wise women and, by corollary, in witchcraft. It is a wound herb and a leaf on a cut will quickly stop bleeding. It is said that Achilles took Chiron the centaur's advice and used it to staunch the wounds of his troops in battle.

In company with elderflower and peppermint it is good for colds and flu. It is also an anti-spasmodic and can have a positive effect on circulatory problems. A child safe remedy in small quantities, but not for use in pregnancy.

Yew
Taxus baccata

A tree that is sacred to pagan Celts and Christians alike. It is slow growing and long-lived, with some individuals thought to be as much as five thousand years old. There is no surprise then that it symbolises eternal life. It is also an extremely poisonous tree, deadly to both people and livestock and is, therefore, also associated with death and mourning.

There is only one part of the tree which is edible, that being the sticky red berry. It is supposed to be very sweet and attracts birds, which void the extremely poisonous green seed, making sure that seedlings are well dispersed. As with many trees, both male and female are needed before berries are formed.

The traditional planting place was a churchyard, although many older yews predate Christianity and must have been associated with pagan sacred sites. This had an added advantage that cattle were unlikely to graze there, and that there was plenty of timber to supply the archers of the Middle Ages.

Yew has recently come to the foreground of plant medicine because it has been discovered that the alkaloid taxol is of value in conventional medicine for treating some forms of cancer.

There is a famous avenue of topiary yew trees in Rutland where the clippings have been harvested for some years. It is good to know that this is of medicinal use.

Bibliography

Anonymous, 1981, *The Wild Flowers of Britain*, Reader's Digest, London.

Beeton, I. M., 1913 (1861), *The Book of Household Management*, Ward Locke & Co, London.

Bown, D., 1995, *Encyclopaedia of Herbs*, Dorling Kindersley, London.

Culpeper, N., 1653, *The British Herbal and Family Physician*, Milner and Company Ltd, London.

Culpeper, N., 1983, *Culpeper's Colour Herbal*, Potterton, D. [ed], Foulsham & Co, London.

David, E., 1966 (1955), *Summer Cooking*, Penguin, London.

Grieve, M., 1994 (1931, revised 1973), *A Modern Herbal*, Leyel, C. F. [ed], Tiger Books International, London.

Griggs, B., 1997 (1981), *New Green Pharmacy*, Vermilion, London.

Kilbracken, J., 1995 (1983), *Easy Way to Wild Flower Recognition*, Kingfisher Books, London.

Mabey, R., 1972, *Food for Free*, Collins, London.

Philips, R. & Foy, N., 1990, *Herbs*, Pan Books, London.

Rhode, E. S., 1969 (1936), *A Garden of Herbs*, Dover, New York.

Uttley, A., 1977 (1931), *The Country Child*, Puffin, London.

INDEX

Knitbone 49
Korean Mint 21

Lamb's Ears 29
Laurel, Bay Sweet 26
Lavender 70
Lavender, Cotton 51
Lawn Chamomile 42
Lemon Balm 23
Lemon Grass 72
Lemon Verbena 72
Leopard's Bane 22
Lesser Calamint 36
Lesser Celandine 38, 39
Lettuce Leaved Basil 24
Lily of the Valley 73
Lincolnshire Spinach 61
Linseed 72
Lovage 73
Lovage, Black 18
Love in Idleness 64

Maidenhair Tree 61
Mallow, Marsh 66
Mallow, Musk 67
Mallow, Wild 67
Marigold, Pot 73
Marjoram, Sweet 74
Marjoram, Wild 74
Marsh Mallow 66
Meadowsweet 74
Meeting Herb 57
Mignonette, Wild 93
Milk Thistle 66
Mint 75
Mint, Korean 21
Miss Jessup's Upright 84
Monk's Pepper 43
Monkshood 15
Mountain Ash 84
Mountain Balm 36
Mugwort 76
Mullein 77
Muscatel Sage 47
Musk Mallow 67
Myrtle 77

Nasturtium 78
Neapolitan Basil 24
Nettle 78

Old Man 76
Onion, Egyptian 46
Onion, Tree 46
Onion, Welsh 46
Oswego Tea 26

Parsley 79
Parsley, Cow 43
Parsley, Flat-leaved 79
Parsley, French 79
Parsley, Hamburg 79
Parsley, Root 79
Pennyroyal 75
Peppermint 75
Pilewort 39
Plantagenet 32
Plantain 79
Pot Marigold 73
Primrose, Evening 56
Primrose, Wild 52
Purple Coneflower 80
Purslane 80

Queen Anne's Lace 43
Queen of the Meadow 74

Red Campion 37
Red Clover 48
Red Robin 65
Red Rose of Lancaster 83
Red Valerian 92
Rhubarb 80
Rhubarb, Chinese 81
Rhubarb, Turkey 81
Ribwort 79
Rocket 81
Rocket, Dyer's 93
Rocket, Wild 81
Roman Chamomile 42
Root Parsley 79
Rose, Apothecary's 83
Rose, Christmas 25

Achillea millefolium 95
Acinos arvensis 25
Aconitum napellus 15
Agastache anethiodora 21
Agastache ragosa 21
Agrimonia eupatoria 16
Ajuga reptans 33
Aloe barbadensis 19
Allium ampeloprasum 60
Allium cepa Proliferum 46
Allium schoenoprasum 46
Allium sativum 60
Allium tuberosum 46
Althea officinalis 66
Althea rosea 66
Anethum graveolens 55
Angelica archangelica 20
Anthemis nobilis
   'Flore Pleno' 41
Anthemis nobilis
   'Treneague' 42
Anthemis tinctoria 41, 42
Anthriscus cerefolium 43
Anthriscus sylvestris 43
Apium graveolens 89
Arctium lappa 34
Armoracia rusticana 68
Arnica montana 22
Artemisia abrotanum 76
Artemisia absinthium 76
Artemisia dracunculus 90
Artemisia vulgaris 76

bacca laurea 27
baccalaureate 27
Bellis perennis 53
Borago officinalis 29
Borago laxifolia 30
Buxus sempervirens 30

Calamintha grandiflora 36
Calamintha nepeta 36
Calendula officinalis 73
Carduus benedictus 66
Carum carvi 37
Cedronella triphylla 22

Centaurium erythraea 40
Centranthus rubra 92
Chelidonium majus 38
Chenopodium bonus
   henricus 61
Cichorium intybus 44
Coriandrum sativum 50
Crataegus laevigata 62
Cytisus scoparius 32

Digitalis purpurea 59

Echinacea purpurea 80
Eruca sativa 81
Eruca vesicaria 81
Eupatorium cannabinum 64

Ficus carica 58
Filipendula ulmaria 74
Foeniculum vulgare 57
Foeniculum vulgare dulce 57

Galega officinalis 61
Galium aparine 47
Galium odoratum 93
genièvre 70
Genista tinctoria 32
Geranium robertianum 65
Gingko biloba 61

Helichrysum italicum 52
Helleborus foetidus 25
Helleborus niger 25
Humulus lupulus 68
Hypericum perforatum 87
Hyssopus officinalis 69, 70

Ilex aquifolium 65
Illicium anisatum 21
Inula helenium 56
Isatis tinctoria 93

jenever 70
Juniperus communis 70

Laurus nobilis 26

103

Lavandula angustifolia 70, 72
Levisticum officinale 73
Linum usitissimum 72, 73
Lippia citriodora 72

Malva moschata 67
Malva sylvestris 67
Marrubium vulgare 69
maythen 41
Melissa officinalis 23
Mentha piperita 75
Mentha pulegium 75
Mentha rotundifolia 75
Mentha spicata 75
Monarda didyma 26
Myrrhis odorata 53
Myrtus communis 77

Nepeta cataria 38
Nepeta glechoma 62
Nepeta mussinii 38

Ocimum basilicum 24
Ocimum sanctum 24
Oenothera biennis 56
Oregano vulgare 74

Pentaglottis sempervirens 19
Petasites hybridus 35
Petroselinum crispum 79
Phuopsis stylosa 94
Pimpinella anisum 21
planta genista 32
Plantago lanceolate 79
Polemonium caeruleum 15
Polemonium reptans 15
Polygonum bistorta 27
Portulaca oleracea 80
Primula veris 51
Primula vulgaris 52

Ranunculus ficaria 39
Resedua lutea 93
Reseda luteola 93
Rheum palmatum 81
Rheum rhaponticum 80

Rosa canina 82
Rosa gallica 83
Rosa gallica 'Versicolor' 83
Rosa rubiginosa 82
Rosa rugosa 83
Rosmarinus officinalis 83
Rumex acetosa 89
Rumex scutatus 90
Ruta graveolens 84

Salvia Icterina 85
Salvia lavandulifolia 85
Salvia officinalis 85
Salvia purpurascens 85
Salvia sclarea 46
Salvia tricolor 85
Salvia verbenaca 47
Sambucus nigra 55
Sanguisorba minor 35
Sanguisorba officinalis 34
Santolina chamaecyparissus 51
Saponaria officinalis 88
Satureja hortensis 87
Satureja montana 87
Sempervivum tectorum 68
Silene vulgaris 36
Silene dioica 37
Silybum marianum 66
Sium sisarum 89
Smyrnium olusatrum 18
Solidago virgaurea 62
Sorbus aucuparia 84
Stachys officinalis 28
Stellaria media 45
Symphytum officinalis 49

Tanacetum balsamita 17
Tanacetum balsamita
   var. tomentosum 17
Tanacetum parthenium 57
Tanacetum vulgare 90
Taraxacum officinale 54
Taxus baccata 95
Thymus vulgaris 91
Trifolium pratense 48
Trifolium repens 48